THE GIRLS' GUIDE TO GROWING UP

Anita Naik
Illustrated by Sarah Horne

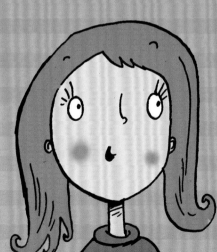

wren
&rook

Contents

What is puberty? 3

Your puberty timeline 4

How do hormones work? 6

Breasts and bras 8

Same age, different stage 10

Skin changes 12

Sweat, smells and personal hygiene 14

Hair in new places 16

Down there 18

What are periods? 20

The practical side of periods 22

Coping with periods 24

Sex explained 26

Making babies 28

New feelings 30

Managing your moods 32

Healthy eating 34

The power of exercise 36

Self-esteem and body image 38

Privacy and your body 40

Puberty for boys 42

Boys have worries, too 44

Words to remember 46

Useful information 47

Index 48

WHAT IS PUBERTY?

In the next few years, you will start to notice some changes happening to your body – both on the outside and the inside!

Puberty is the name given to the stage in your life when you change from being a girl to being a woman. It sounds quite weird but it's actually amazing!

Puberty can start when girls are anywhere between 8 and 13 years old, and sometimes older. It doesn't happen overnight – it's a slow process. Eventually everything from your height to your body shape will be affected – your face might even change a bit!

The purpose of puberty is to get your body ready to have a baby when you're older, if you decide you want one.

Sometimes going through puberty can make you feel shy or embarrassed, but there's no need to be – it's a normal and natural process.

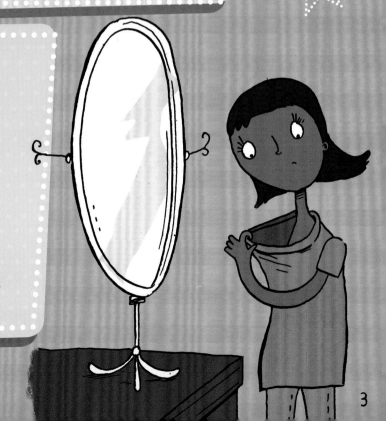

YOUR PUBERTY TIMELINE

Your body has its own unique internal clock, and it will only start puberty when it's ready. However, this is a rough guide to what will happen to your body and when.

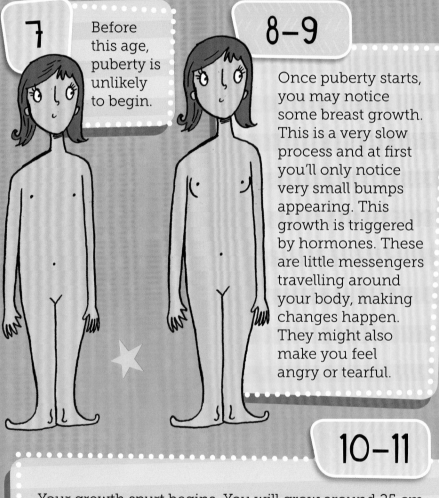

7 Before this age, puberty is unlikely to begin.

8–9 Once puberty starts, you may notice some breast growth. This is a very slow process and at first you'll only notice very small bumps appearing. This growth is triggered by hormones. These are little messengers travelling around your body, making changes happen. They might also make you feel angry or tearful.

10–11 Your growth spurt begins. You will grow around 25 cm between now and the start of your first period. After your first period, you will grow about another 5 cm. Your body will also start to change shape at this time. Your hips will widen, and your thighs and bottom will get bigger.

11–12

Your breasts will continue to develop; this process carries on until you're around 17. Your period will start some time around the age of 11, though it can be earlier or later. You may notice that spots come and go on your face around your period.

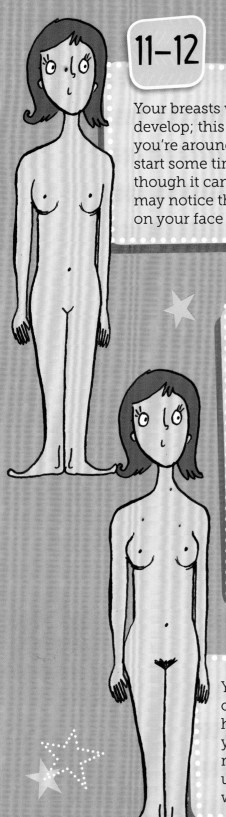

12–13

Body hair will start to grow between your legs and under your arms. The hair on your legs may thicken or darken. This process sometimes begins before your breasts start to grow. You may also notice a smell, known as body odour, when you're doing sport or when the weather is hot. This is caused by sweat mixing with bacteria on your skin.

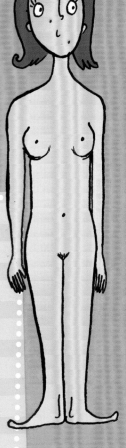

14–18

Your period will begin if it hasn't already, or it may settle into a regular cycle. Your height and weight will keep changing and your breasts will continue to grow. Your moods may vary a lot, and spots may crop up. It sounds exhausting, but becoming a woman is actually pretty exciting!

HOW DO HORMONES WORK?

During puberty, your hormones tell your body what to do.

Hormones are chemical messengers that travel around your body, starting each stage of the puberty journey.

A part of the brain called the hypothalamus makes GnRH.

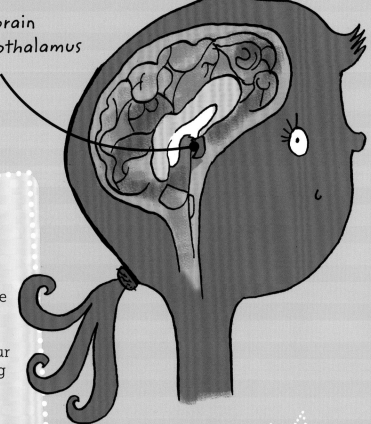

At around the age of 8, your brain starts to make a hormone called GnRH, which then triggers two more hormones to be made in the brain. It's these hormones that tell your ovaries to start making female sex hormones called oestrogen and progesterone, which then kickstart puberty.

Oestrogen prompts your breasts to start growing. It also starts the process that makes parts of your body ready to have a baby, such as your uterus (or womb), where a baby grows, and your Fallopian tubes, which carry your eggs to your womb. Oestrogen also plays a role in your growth spurt, helping to make you a more curvy, womanly shape. The other sex hormone, progesterone, helps your periods to begin, because it thickens the lining of the uterus each month.

There's a lot of talk about hormones being female or male, but boys and girls actually have both sets. Boys have some female hormones and girls have some male hormones, such as testosterone, which is needed for muscle and bone growth.

Why do my feelings seem different?

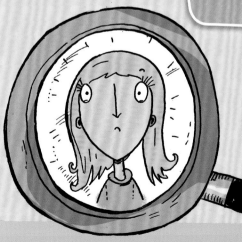

As these hormones travel around your body, they can start to play havoc with your emotions. This is normal, and as puberty goes on, these surges settle down until you hardly notice them.

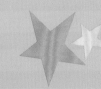

BREASTS AND BRAS

Budding breasts, as they are known when they begin to grow, are often the first sign that you're entering puberty.

Breast growth usually starts when you are between about 9 and 12 years old. Breasts take a long time to grow, and even as long as five years to mature fully.

At first, budding breasts look like a small, raised bump under each of your nipples. These buds will gradually grow and change shape. At the same time, your nipples and the surrounding skin, called areolas, will also get bigger and slightly darker. When they are fully grown, your breasts will be round with the areolas and nipples becoming small mounds that sit on top.

During puberty, you may find that your breasts start to feel sore. This tenderness is a sign that they are getting bigger, and you may need to give them some support. A training bra may help. These are soft bras that gently support your breast area. They look just like crop tops. When you feel ready, perhaps go shopping with a parent, older sister or older friend so they can help you find a first bra that is comfortable.

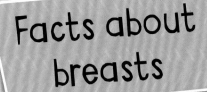

Facts about breasts

★ Breasts come in many sizes and shapes, and nipples vary in colour.

★ You can't force your breasts to grow faster, or get bigger or smaller, by doing activities or exercises. They are unique to you and grow in their own time.

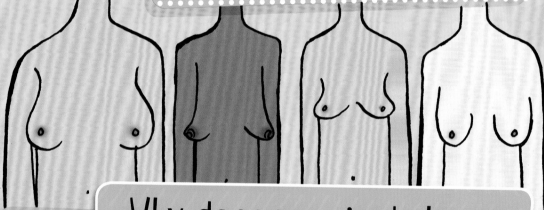

Why does my nipple have a dent in it?

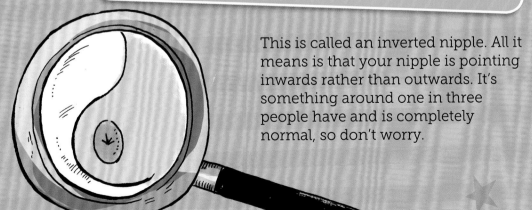

This is called an inverted nipple. All it means is that your nipple is pointing inwards rather than outwards. It's something around one in three people have and is completely normal, so don't worry.

SAME AGE, DIFFERENT STAGE

One of the amazing parts of puberty is that you and your friends can be the same age but look and feel very different.

Our bodies have their own unique routes through puberty. This is why some of your friends may suddenly seem curvy, others will shoot upwards and some will remain small. Everyone's body is different in height, weight, hairiness and breast size.

It can make you feel uncomfortable about yourself if you're the first to grow tall or the last to have breasts. Remember that puberty is not a race. The way you look today isn't the way you will look by the end of puberty. Relax and let things happen at their own pace.

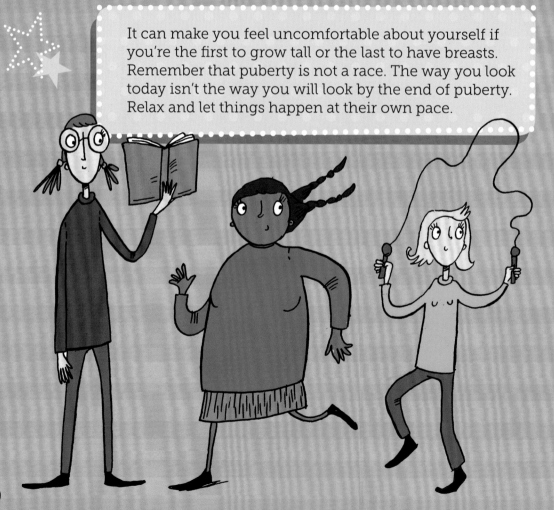

How much you grow depends on your genes – the physical traits you inherited from your mum and dad. So if you want a rough idea of how you might look at the end of puberty, look at the height of women on both your mum's and dad's sides of your family.

What to expect

★ At around 9 years old, you may become much taller quite quickly.

★ Your arms and legs will grow before the rest of your body.

★ Most girls reach the peak of their height growth about six months before their first period. If you suddenly shoot up in height, you might soon start your period.

Why do I weigh more?

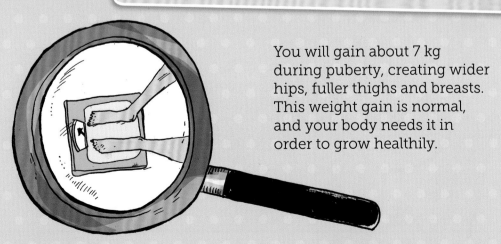

You will gain about 7 kg during puberty, creating wider hips, fuller thighs and breasts. This weight gain is normal, and your body needs it in order to grow healthily.

SKIN CHANGES

Nothing announces that you're growing up faster than a few spots appearing on your skin.

They can be a pain, but there are lots of ways to manage spots.

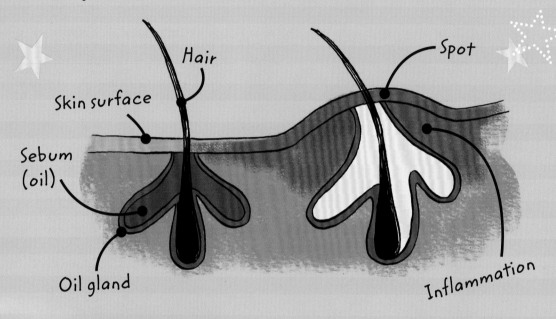

Hair

Spot

Skin surface

Sebum (oil)

Oil gland

Inflammation

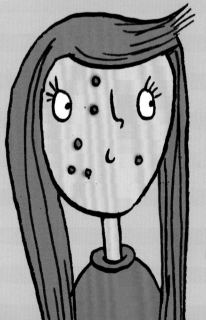

Acne is a skin condition that causes different kinds of spots on the skin. It is triggered by testosterone, the male hormone that surges around your body during puberty. It makes your glands produce too much oil, which then blocks the tiny openings in your skin called pores. The oil mixes with bacteria and becomes a spot.

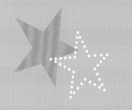

Certain factors can affect how and when you get spots during puberty. Surging levels of hormones at the start of your period can cause an outbreak, and genetics come into play again: if your parents had spots during puberty, it's likely that you will too.

Tips to fight spots

★ Don't pick or pop them. This will make the bacteria spread and your spots will last longer.

★ Talk to a pharmacist about the best products for your skin. Use a product for at least four weeks before deciding whether it works or not.

★ Doctors will take spots seriously if you have a bad outbreak. If they're getting you down, visit your GP to discuss medication that may help.

What are these stretch marks?

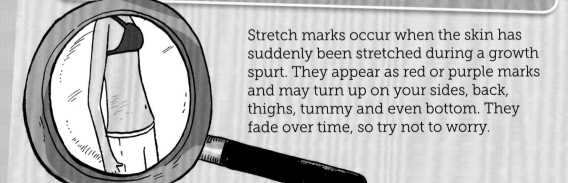

Stretch marks occur when the skin has suddenly been stretched during a growth spurt. They appear as red or purple marks and may turn up on your sides, back, thighs, tummy and even bottom. They fade over time, so try not to worry.

SWEAT, SMELLS AND PERSONAL HYGIENE

Our bodies are covered in glands that release sweat to cool us down when we're hot. You're unlikely to have noticed your sweat much as a child, but during puberty you will.

Puberty revs up your sweat glands, making them more active. You'll start to notice that you and your friends sweat more. You'll see it on your face, feel it under your arms and, on hot days, you may find it trickling down your skin.

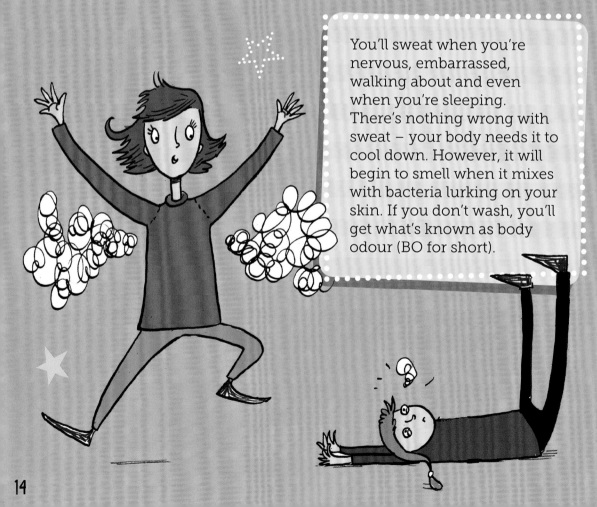

You'll sweat when you're nervous, embarrassed, walking about and even when you're sleeping. There's nothing wrong with sweat – your body needs it to cool down. However, it will begin to smell when it mixes with bacteria lurking on your skin. If you don't wash, you'll get what's known as body odour (BO for short).

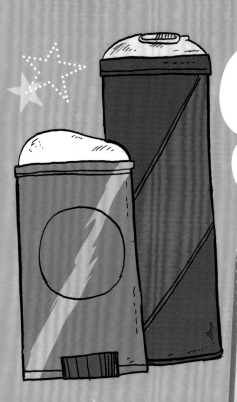

It's normal to sweat a bit more when:
★ you feel hot
★ you eat spicy foods
★ you exercise
★ you are angry or anxious
★ you are nearing your period

The best way to get rid of body odour is to practise good personal hygiene. This means washing daily, changing into clean clothes every day and perhaps choosing to use a deodorant or antiperspirant product under your arms. Antiperspirants reduce the amount of sweat that comes to the surface, and can also prevent BO.

Why do I feel sweaty down below?

Just like your underarms, your genitals will get sweaty and smell bad if you don't wash them every day. However, this sensitive area does not need deodorant – soap and water is fine.

HAIR IN NEW PLACES

When you find new fuzz, don't worry. Discovering new body hair is part of the adventure during puberty!

Where once your skin was smooth, you will gradually start to see hair growing under your arms and between your legs. The hair on your legs and arms may thicken or darken too. If you're worrying that body hair will appear overnight, don't panic. Hair growth at puberty starts very slowly.

At first, the hair that grows under your arms and in the pubic region between your legs is soft and downy, and you may find you feel a bit itchy. However, this will pass and the hair will become curlier, thicker and darker.

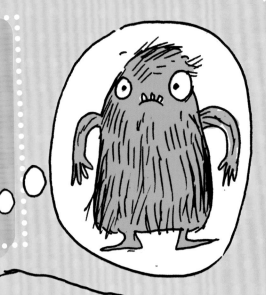

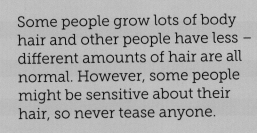

Some people grow lots of body hair and other people have less – different amounts of hair are all normal. However, some people might be sensitive about their hair, so never tease anyone.

Body hair is amazing! It helps keep your body temperature at a constant level, which is especially important during puberty. It does this by helping to hold on to heat when you are cold, and taking sweat away from your skin when you are hot. Body hair also helps to protect some of your most sensitive areas.

You may notice that some older girls choose to shave or wax their underarm or leg hair. There are no health reasons to do this, so chat to your parents or older sister to help you choose what's right for you.

Facts about body hair

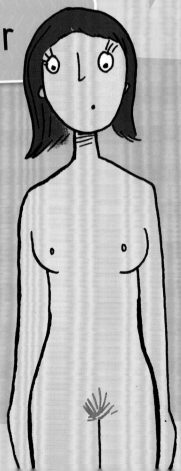

★ Hair growth varies on different parts of your body. For example, the hair between your legs will stay quite short, but your head hair can grow very long.

★ Body hair can be a different colour to the hair on your head. Your body hair's colour will depend on ethnic factors, like where your family is from.

DOWN THERE

There are female sex organs on both the inside and outside of your body, and some of them change during puberty too.

Knowing about them will help you to understand the changes that happen to your body during puberty.

On the inside

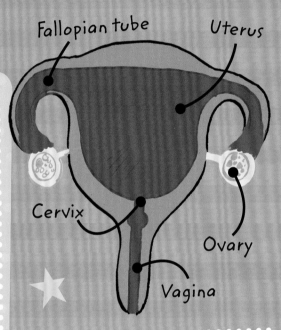

Fallopian tube · Uterus · Cervix · Ovary · Vagina

Ovaries

Most girls have two ovaries. These grow to the size of walnuts during puberty. Your ovaries have been storing eggs ever since you were born. At puberty, hormones signal one egg each month to start maturing and be released from an ovary. This process is known as ovulation.

Fallopian tubes

These tubes connect your ovaries to the uterus. The egg travels through one of the tubes during ovulation.

Uterus (womb)

This is the pear-shaped organ where a baby grows. It stretches naturally as the baby gets bigger.

Cervix

The narrow opening at the bottom of the uterus.

Vagina

This muscular tube goes from your uterus to the outside of your body. It has very stretchy walls, because a baby travels down it to be born.

On the outside

Your outer sex organs are known as the vulva.

Vaginal opening
This is the opening to your vagina. During puberty, the area around the opening becomes covered with pubic hair.

Hymen
A thin layer of skin called the hymen covers your vaginal opening when you are born. You can't see it, and as you grow older, it thins and wears away.

Outer and inner labia
The labia are folds of skin that protect your vaginal opening. These get larger during puberty as the rest of your body grows.

Clitoris
The small pea-shaped lump at the top of your labia is called the clitoris. It is very sensitive to touch.

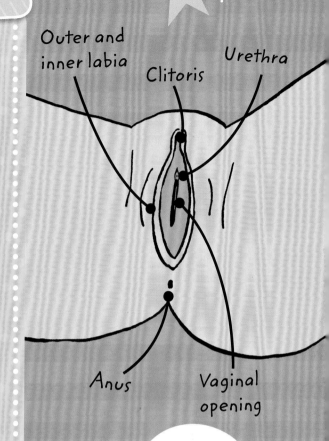

Outer and inner labia

Clitoris

Urethra

Anus

Vaginal opening

Your wee, or urine, comes out of the end of a tube called the urethra. Your poo, or faeces, leaves your body through a hole called the anus. These parts aren't really affected by puberty, but getting to know your body is an important part of growing up.

WHAT ARE PERIODS?

Periods are a normal and natural bodily function, but they are a big change to get used to. It's useful to learn about periods to help you get ready and know how to deal with them.

Your periods start when your body recognises that you have developed enough to have a baby one day.

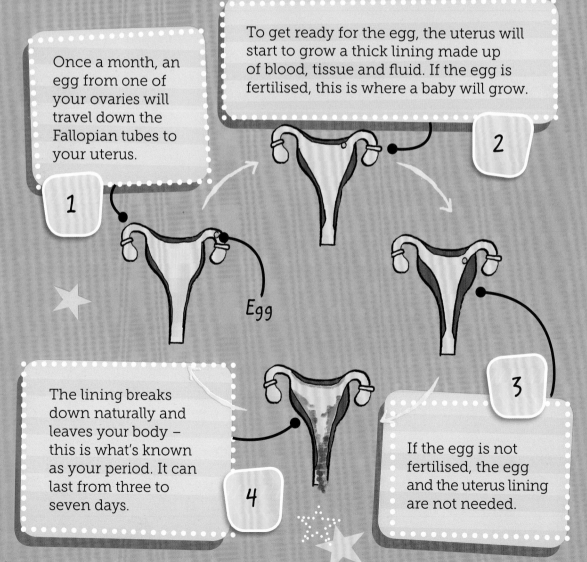

To get ready for the egg, the uterus will start to grow a thick lining made up of blood, tissue and fluid. If the egg is fertilised, this is where a baby will grow.

2

Once a month, an egg from one of your ovaries will travel down the Fallopian tubes to your uterus.

1

Egg

If the egg is not fertilised, the egg and the uterus lining are not needed.

3

The lining breaks down naturally and leaves your body – this is what's known as your period. It can last from three to seven days.

4

Remember, you are not ill when you have your period, even though there is blood. It is a natural female function that will happen every month until you are in your fifties (unless you are pregnant). Some girls find the idea of periods a bit upsetting at first. If that's you, talk to someone about how you feel. It's a normal and natural part of life, so ask your mum, aunt or big sister about it.

Another word for a period is 'menstruation'. It's a longer word that means the same thing!

How much blood will I lose?

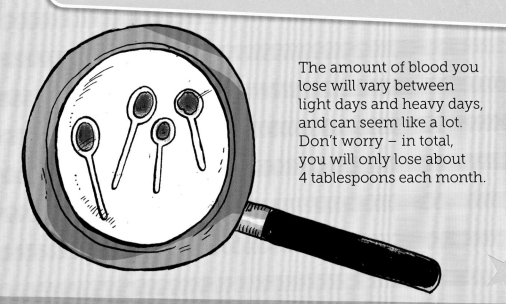

The amount of blood you lose will vary between light days and heavy days, and can seem like a lot. Don't worry – in total, you will only lose about 4 tablespoons each month.

THE PRACTICAL SIDE OF PERIODS

One of the trickiest parts of having your period is dealing with the blood flow.

Periods start off slowly, get a little heavier in days two and three, then slow down and stop. There are two main products you can use to help manage the blood flow.

Sanitary towels

Sanitary towels are absorbent pads that soak up the flow of blood from your period. They have a sticky back that attaches to the inside of your knickers, so they are comfortable and easily disposable. They come in different thicknesses and sizes for lighter and heavier flow days. Sanitary towels need to be changed frequently to make sure blood doesn't soak through.

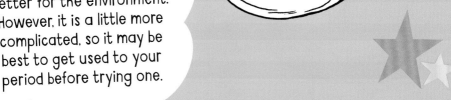

Another period product is the menstrual cup, which is better for the environment. However, it is a little more complicated, so it may be best to get used to your period before trying one.

Tampons

Tampons are cylinders of absorbent material that fit inside your vagina and soak up the blood. Once the tampon is in, you don't feel it at all, and you don't feel fluid coming out of you. Tampons come in different absorbencies, and some have applicators to make inserting them easier.

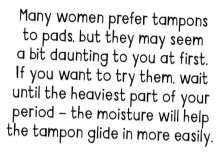

Many women prefer tampons to pads, but they may seem a bit daunting to you at first. If you want to try them, wait until the heaviest part of your period – the moisture will help the tampon glide in more easily.

Start with a small size and follow the instructions in the box. If it doesn't work the first time, don't worry. Being nervous or tense can make it more difficult, so just relax and try again later.

Can tampons get lost in my body?

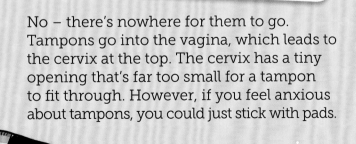

No – there's nowhere for them to go. Tampons go into the vagina, which leads to the cervix at the top. The cervix has a tiny opening that's far too small for a tampon to fit through. However, if you feel anxious about tampons, you could just stick with pads.

COPING WITH PERIODS

You might have heard stories about how difficult and painful periods are. Try not to worry about what others say.

Everyone finds their own way of managing their periods so they are easier to cope with.

Working out your menstrual cycle

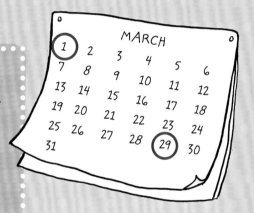

Your period comes about every 28 days, or four weeks. This time is known as your menstrual cycle. The cycle begins when your period starts, so counting 28 days forward from then will help you predict when your next period will begin. However, during puberty, you may find you have bigger or smaller gaps between your periods. By the end of puberty they will have fallen into a more regular pattern.

Cramps and pains

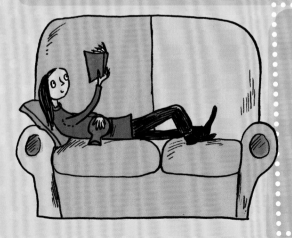

When you have your period, the muscly walls of your uterus help to get rid of the blood by squeezing or contracting. These are known as menstrual cramps and can hurt, but they are normal and help your body. To reduce cramps, put a hot water bottle on your tummy or go for a walk. Painkillers can help, so ask your parents for advice.

Period myths

✗ "Other people can tell when you are on your period."

False: no one will know unless you tell them.

✗ "You can't do sport when you have a period."

False: you can do any sport you enjoy. The only activity that needs more preparation is swimming, when you would need to use a tampon.

✗ "Your period stops in water."

False: your period carries on if you have a bath or go swimming, so use tampons to stay clean in the pool.

Three out of four women get some form of PMS.

Why do I feel up and down around my period?

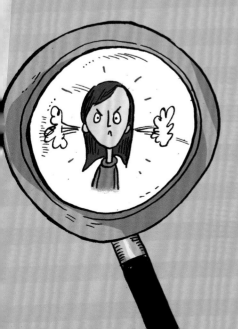

The changing levels of hormones around your period can cause emotional symptoms (like grumpiness, sadness and tearfulness) and physical ones (like spots, cramps or headaches). This is known as premenstrual syndrome, or 'PMS'.

Symptoms can appear up to five days before your period starts, and may disappear during your period. If you're feeling down, try treating yourself to something you enjoy, and take it easy until your period is over.

SEX EXPLAINED

Having babies is probably the furthest thing from your mind during puberty, but it's important to know how they are made.

Sexual intercourse – known as sex – is how babies are made, and it's what your body is preparing for during puberty.

Lots of people find the whole topic of sex very embarrassing to discuss or even say, but sex is a normal activity between adult people who love and care about each other.

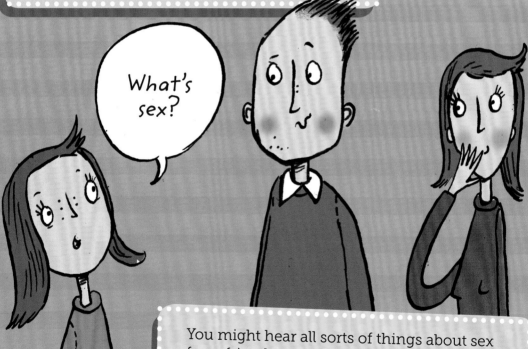

What's sex?

You might hear all sorts of things about sex from friends at school, but they're often not true. If you have questions, ask a parent or a grown-up you trust. The back of this book also lists some useful websites.

During sex, two people kiss, cuddle and get sexually excited. When a man is excited, his penis gets hard, or erect. When a woman is excited, her vagina releases a slippery fluid.

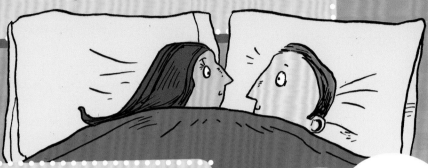

When a man and a woman have sex, the man's penis goes into the woman's vagina. When the man reaches the peak of excitement, he releases a small amount of a fluid called semen. This process is known as ejaculation. Semen contains millions of sperm, the male sex cell. The sperm swim into the woman's body and try to reach an egg.

Sex isn't just about making babies. It's also something adults do when they love each other, because it's a way for them to show affection and to feel good. See the next page for how people can choose to have sex without making babies.

What if I think sex sounds scary?

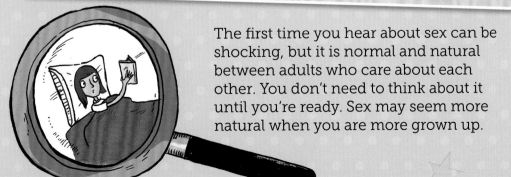

The first time you hear about sex can be shocking, but it is normal and natural between adults who care about each other. You don't need to think about it until you're ready. Sex may seem more natural when you are more grown up.

MAKING BABIES

Making a baby may seem very mysterious, but it is important to understand what your body can do.

To make a baby, sperm from a man's body has to meet and join with an egg from a woman's body.

How is a baby made?

If a male sperm joins with a female egg after sex, it is called fertilisation. If this happens, the egg becomes an embryo, which nestles in the woman's uterus where it will grow to become a baby. This means the woman is pregnant, so her periods will stop because the lining of the uterus is needed.

Female egg

Male sperm

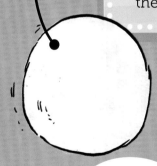

When adults don't want to make babies, they use what's known as contraception. This describes a variety of methods that either prevent the sperm from meeting the egg or stop the egg from being fertilised.

Pregnancy

Pregnancy is the time when a baby is growing inside the mother. It lasts 9 months, in which time the embryo becomes a baby. The growing child stretches the uterus, which is why the mother develops a large pregnancy bump.

Labour

The process of giving birth is known as labour. A baby can arrive by vaginal delivery, where the woman pushes the baby out through her vagina, or by a method called a caesarean section, when doctors cut the woman's uterus in surgery to get the baby out.

NEW FEELINGS

Puberty has a lot to answer for if you find your moods changing all the time during puberty.

Growing up can be hard. You may start to feel attracted to other people, and hormones surging around your body can give you mixed emotions.

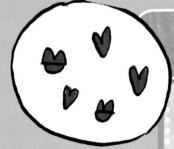

Special feelings

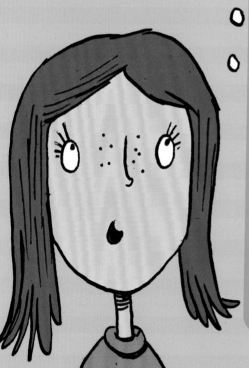

It's perfectly normal to start thinking about sex a lot more during puberty, and some girls find that they start becoming attracted to people they never thought about before: perhaps a boy who lives nearby, or a girl they get on with really well. If this happens to you, you might start to imagine kissing or touching them. These thoughts are a safe way to explore your new feelings, but don't let anyone pressure you into dating or kissing someone before you're ready. You might also find that you are not attracted to anyone. This is normal too, and you shouldn't feel worried about it.

Mood swings

Moody, sulky, stroppy, angry, tearful, sleepy and cheeky —they may sound like Snow White's seven dwarfs, but they're just some of the emotions you might feel during puberty. The process of growing up can be tough sometimes, and it might make you feel confused, angry and upset all at the same time. Hormones also change how you feel, sometimes making you tired, tearful and over-sensitive. No wonder people say moods and puberty seem to go hand in hand!

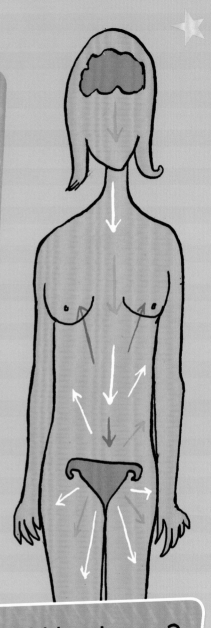

If you imagine all the hormones flooding your body during puberty, it's easier to understand why your emotions might sometimes feel all over the place.

When will my moods settle down?

One of the roles of the hormones testosterone and oestrogen is to rewire the emotional areas of the brain. Your mood swings will even out as soon as the hormones have done their job.

MANAGING YOUR MOODS

**Sometimes you won't know how to handle
your changing emotions: that's okay.**

During puberty you will learn to cope with intense emotions, just as it
will take time to get to know your new body. Here's what will help –
and what won't!

Talk about how you feel

This can be hard, because sometimes you don't actually know how
you feel! Remember, you don't have to spill your heart out. Just
tell others you feel low or emotional, and tell them what you need
– even if it's just a bit of time out. Be honest when you feel cranky
and upset. Trying to put on a brave face, or marching around being
cross at everyone, will just lead to more bad feelings.

Chat to your parents

Parents aren't mind-
readers – they won't know
if you're sad, upset or have
had a bad day unless you
say so. They'll understand
that sometimes you'll
need time alone and
sometimes you'll want
a hug of reassurance.

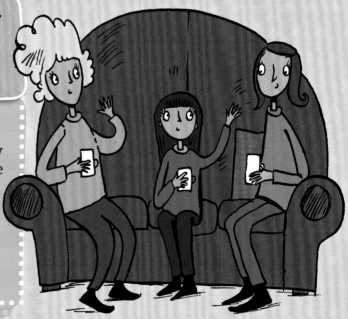

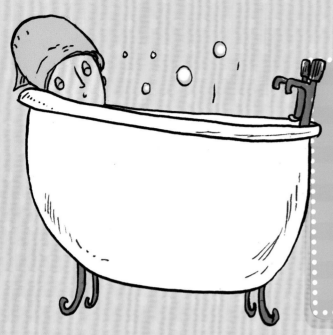

Relax

This doesn't mean spending hours on your phone or with friends, but really taking time to chill out. Puberty takes a lot of energy, and at times you are going to feel exhausted and fed up. It's really important to spend some of your time winding down.

What won't help my mood swings?

★ **A bad diet:** eating badly or skipping meals during puberty will give you less energy. Tiredness can lead to mood swings and arguments.

★ **Keeping your feelings locked up inside:** hiding how you're feeling will only make you more angry and sad.

★ **A lack of sleep:** without 10 hours of sleep a night, it's hard to control your emotions.

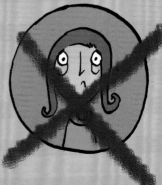

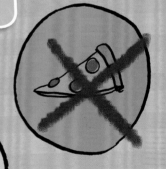

HEALTHY EATING

Eating well during puberty is vital if you want to feel good. Healthy food will help you to have fewer mood swings and allow your body to develop properly.

As you grow older, you can choose your own food more and more, especially when you're out and about. The urge to eat fast food or junk food can be strong.

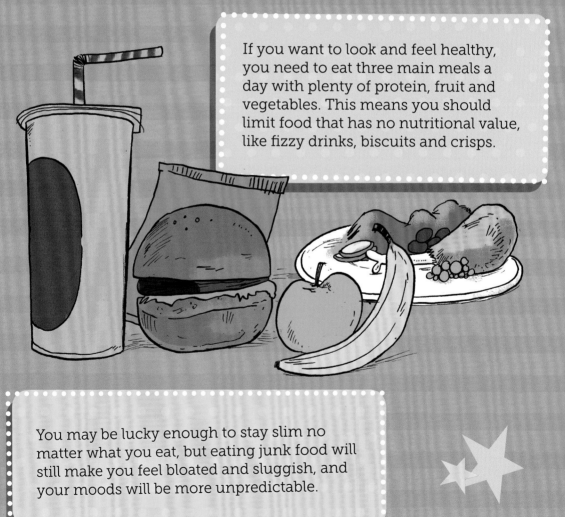

If you want to look and feel healthy, you need to eat three main meals a day with plenty of protein, fruit and vegetables. This means you should limit food that has no nutritional value, like fizzy drinks, biscuits and crisps.

You may be lucky enough to stay slim no matter what you eat, but eating junk food will still make you feel bloated and sluggish, and your moods will be more unpredictable.

> To support the large increases in your height during puberty, you will become more hungry and will need to eat larger portions.

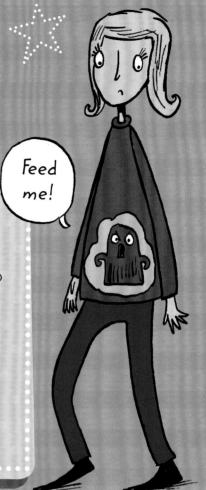

Feed me!

At puberty, some girls don't like seeing their bodies putting on fat and becoming curvier. While these changes are normal, it can lead some girls to think they have to diet or skip meals.

Don't get sucked into the idea that you have to be worried about what you eat and what you weigh. If you're concerned about your weight, speak to your parents and see your doctor for proper advice. Trying trendy diets that your friends are on can be bad for your health.

What do I do if I think my friend has an eating disorder?

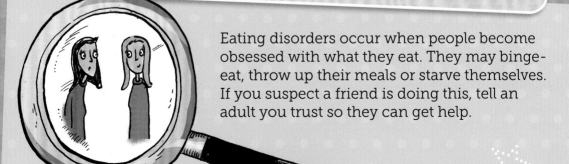

Eating disorders occur when people become obsessed with what they eat. They may binge-eat, throw up their meals or starve themselves. If you suspect a friend is doing this, tell an adult you trust so they can get help.

THE POWER OF EXERCISE

Being active is an important part of staying healthy during puberty.

If you're fit and energetic, you'll feel better and will also have more body confidence.

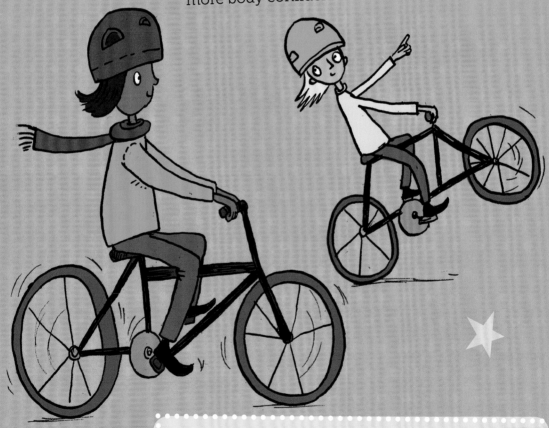

Exercise does a number of things during puberty. It helps you stay at a healthy weight, reduces stress, makes you sleep better and gives you more energy. It also increases your muscle and bone strength, and keeps your heart healthy.

Unfortunately, studies show that some girls get less active as puberty progresses. Much of this is down to feeling self-conscious, hating PE or being embarrassed when getting changed for sport.

An hour sounds a lot, but it's not if you break it up:

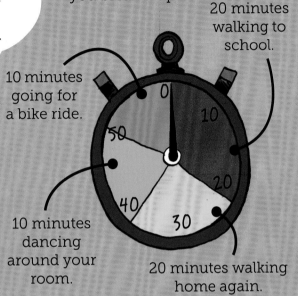

20 minutes walking to school.

10 minutes going for a bike ride.

Even if you're not the captain of a school team, it's easy to stay active. Just make sure you exercise for 30 to 60 minutes a day, whether that's cycling to school, running for the bus or doing an activity like swimming.

10 minutes dancing around your room.

20 minutes walking home again.

Which exercise is best for me?

During puberty your body is changing, so try plenty of different activities to see what suits you best. If team sports like hockey aren't for you, why not go for:

★ ice skating
★ dancing
★ running
★ swimming

★ cycling
★ martial arts
★ skateboarding
★ rock climbing

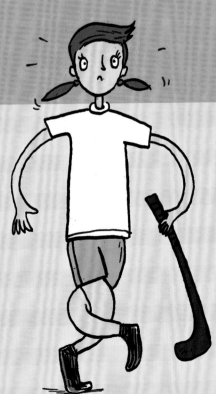

SELF-ESTEEM AND BODY IMAGE

How we feel about ourselves is known as self-esteem.

Your own self-esteem can affect the way you behave and how you think about your body, so it's important to look after your well-being.

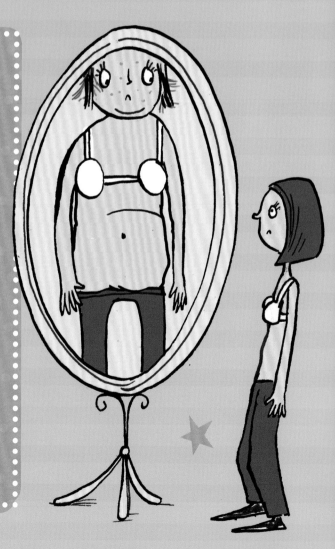

'Body image' means how you see yourself, and it takes time to come to terms with while everything is changing. Perhaps you feel you're too tall or too short, too spotty or too greasy. One thing is almost guaranteed: you'll imagine things are worse than they actually are.

When you're feeling low, remember: the way you look today is not what you'll look like at the end of puberty.

Also bear in mind that you are still the same person as before. How tall you are, how big your breasts may be or how much you weigh does not define who you are.

To feel better about yourself, try these top tips:

★ Think about what you're good at, from being kind to being great at art or sport. Focus on the positives.

★ Don't waste time comparing yourself to others; this is a recipe for misery.

★ If you feel low, tell someone. Talking really helps.

★ Work out what saps your confidence. Is it a friend who says mean things, programmes you watch or what you read on social media? Whatever it is, avoid it.

★ Believe in yourself. Don't talk yourself out of things before you even try. This is low self-esteem talking.

★ Take the focus off celebrities – they aren't helpful role models when you're feeling down and going through puberty.

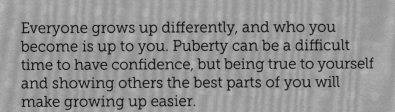

Everyone grows up differently, and who you become is up to you. Puberty can be a difficult time to have confidence, but being true to yourself and showing others the best parts of you will make growing up easier.

PRIVACY AND YOUR BODY

During puberty you'll start to feel the need for more privacy.

Part of growing up and becoming an independent person is choosing what you want to tell or show to other people.

Needing privacy means you may not want to tell your parents everything you're thinking and feeling, like you did as a kid. You also may not want to spend as much time with them. This is normal behaviour and not something to be worried about. Talk to your parents and tell them what you need and why, so they can help make life easier for you at home.

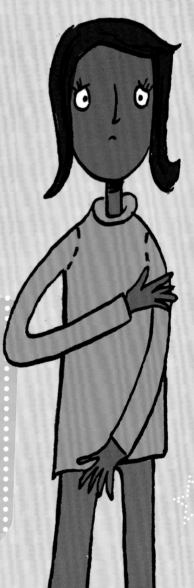

You may also start to feel that you want to keep your body more private and may not want to get changed in front of others. You might also find that you hate comments other people make about your body, and get angry and upset when they talk about 'How you've grown!' or 'How big you're getting!'

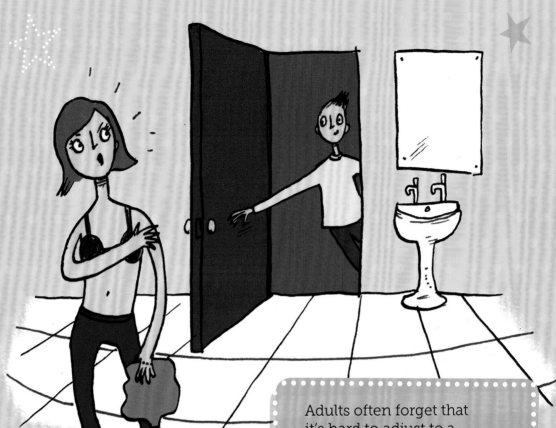

Your genital area is private. No one should ask to see or touch your sex organs, or ask you to look at or touch anyone else's. There may be times, however, when you should show your parents or doctor if you have worries about your body.

Adults often forget that it's hard to adjust to a new body shape without becoming sensitive about it, so if you don't like family members drawing attention to your body, tell them so. The same goes for more privacy. You might need to remind people – especially your parents – that you are changing and don't always want siblings in the bathroom when you're having a wash.

PUBERTY FOR BOYS

Boys do not have periods, but they go through puberty too.

Like girls, the changes will affect every boy differently.
Boys usually start puberty later than girls, so some of the boys
you know may be shorter or look younger than girls.

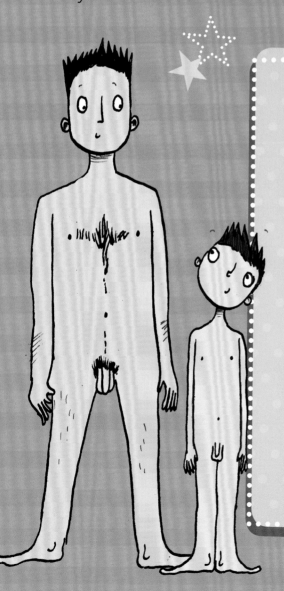

From around 12 years old
(sometimes older, sometimes
younger), boys experience
changes inside and outside
their bodies that are triggered
by sex hormones, especially
testosterone. This causes:

★ a growth spurt that makes
   them bigger and taller, and
   more muscular.

★ the growth of facial and
   pubic hair, plus more hair
   on their bodies.

★ their voice to get deeper.

★ their sex organs to get
   bigger, and their testicles
   to start producing sperm.

★ erections (when their penis
   gets hard), sometimes for
   no reason at all.

The reason a boy's voice gets deeper at puberty is that his voice box grows and tilts forward. This gives boys a visible lump in the throat, known as an Adam's apple.

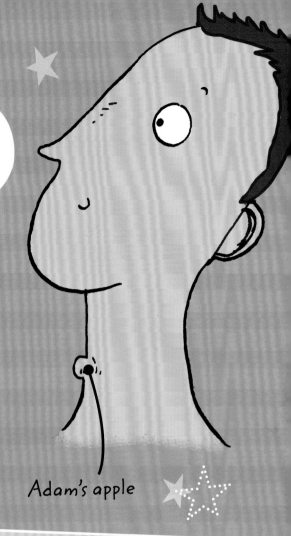

Adam's apple

All these things happen slowly, but the growth stage in boys is more rapid than it is in girls. Girls grow about 5 cm a year during their growth spurt, but boys can shoot up twice as much! This means some boys go through a stage where they look tall and gangly.

Why do boys have such big feet?

Our bodies don't grow neatly. The bones that grow first in boys during puberty are the ones in their feet.

BOYS HAVE WORRIES, TOO

You may feel that boys are like an alien species during puberty.

Since they don't have periods, you may think boys have it easy growing up, but that couldn't be further from the truth.

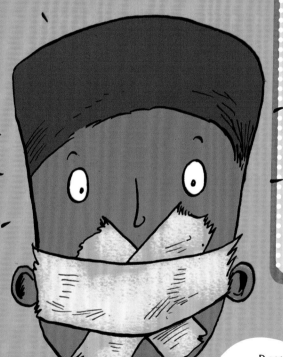

Like girls, boys go through a whole host of physical and emotional changes that leave them feeling vulnerable and worried. However, boys can sometimes feel more pressure than girls to put on a brave face as they grow up. This means many don't tell anyone how they feel, so their thoughts and worries stay in their heads and get them down.

Boys tend to get more spots than girls, as they have a larger amount of the male sex hormone testosterone. They might get spots on their faces, chests or backs, making them feel self-conscious and unconfident.

Some people think that all men should be big and strong, so being small or the last to hit puberty can be tough. However, boys shouldn't be made to feel in any hurry to grow taller or stronger. Puberty takes its time for both boys and girls.

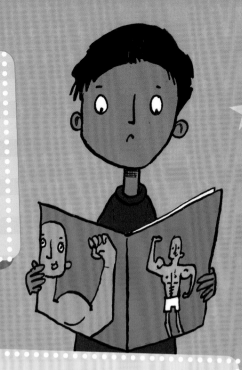

Don't imagine that you're the only one going through a difficult time at puberty. Boys need as much understanding and kindness as girls do. You can help by not making fun of their changing voices, their rapid growth spurts or their newly growing facial hair.

Why am I taller than all the boys?

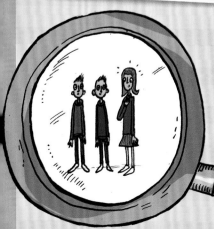

Girls start puberty before boys. Girls have their growth spurt when they're around 10 years old, whilst boys have theirs around 12. This means that girls tower above boys for a few years. By 14, the boys will have caught up and many will be taller than you.

Words to remember

acne A skin condition that causes lots of spots.

body odour (BO) A smell that occurs when sweat contacts bacteria on the skin.

cervix The neck of the uterus or womb.

contraception A range of methods that prevent pregnancy.

egg The female sex cell produced in the ovaries. It is needed to make a baby.

fertilisation When a male sperm joins with a female egg.

genitals The reproductive organs of men or women.

hormones Chemical messengers that cause a change in the body.

labia Folds of skin that cover the opening of a woman's vagina.

menstruation Also known as a **period**, this is the monthly bleed that occurs when the lining of the uterus is shed.

oestrogen One of the female sex hormones.

ovary The place where eggs are stored. Girls have two of them.

ovulation The release of an egg from the ovaries midway through a menstrual cycle.

penis The male sex organ through which urine and sperm leave the body.

pregnancy The period of nine months in which a baby develops inside a woman's uterus.

progesterone One of the female sex hormones.

semen A mixture of sperm and fluid. The fluid allows the sperm to swim.

sperm The male sex cell produced in the testicles. It is needed to make a baby.

testicles Also known as balls, these are where sperm cells are made.

testosterone The main male sex hormone.

uterus Also known as the **womb**, this is where a baby grows and develops until birth.

vagina The muscular tube that leads from the uterus to the outside of the body.

Useful information

BBC	http://tinyurl.org/sex-stis/puberty	Sexual health site that includes information about puberty.
Beat	0345 634 7650 www.b-eat.co.uk	Support and help for eating disorders.
Becoming a Teen	www.becomingateen.co.uk	Information about puberty, periods and products from tampon-makers Lil-Lets.
Being Girl	www.beinggirl.co.uk	Puberty and relationship advice from the makers of Tampax and Always sanitary products.
Childline	0800 1111 www.childline.org.uk	Help and advice for kids and teens from a confidential counsellor.
Family Lives	0808 800 2222 www.familylives.org.uk	An advice organisation for parents and kids covering all areas of family life, including puberty.
NHS	http://tinyurl.com/z89nyoa	The NHS puberty information page, full of useful facts.
Tampax	www.tampax.co.uk	Advice and tips on periods and puberty from Tampax.

Index

Acne	12, 44
Baby / Babies	3, 7, 18, 20, 26–29
Body hair	5, 16–17
Breasts	5, 7–11, 38
Confidence	36, 39
Contraception	27, 28
Cramps	24–25
Diet	33, 35
Egg	7, 18, 20, 27, 28
Erection	27, 42
Exercise	9, 15, 36–37
Feelings	7, 30, 32–33
Genital(s)	15, 19, 41
Growth spurt	4, 7, 13, 42–43, 45
Healthy eating	34–35
Height	3, 5, 10–11, 35
Hormones	6–7, 12–13, 25, 30–31, 42, 44

Menstruation	21 (see also: Periods)
Mood	5, 30–34
Penis	27, 42
Periods	4–5, 7, 11, 13, 15, 20–25, 28
Pregnancy	27, 29
Premenstrual syndrome (PMS)	25
Pubic hair	16–17, 19, 42
Sanitary towels	22
Self-esteem	38–39
Sex	26–28, 30
Spots	5, 12–13, 25, 44
Sweat	5, 14–15, 17
Tampons	23, 25
Uterus	7, 18, 20, 24, 28–29
Vagina	18–19, 23, 27, 29
Weight	5, 10–11, 35, 36

First published in Great Britain in 2016 by Wayland
This edition published in 2017 by Wren & Rook

Copyright © Hodder and Stoughton Limited, 2016

All rights reserved.

Editor: Liza Miller
Design: Collaborate Agency
Illustration: Sarah Horne, Advocate Art

ISBN: 978 1 5263 6018 2
20 19 18 17 16 15 14 13

Wren & Rook
An imprint of
Hachette Children's Group
Part of Hodder & Stoughton
Carmelite House
50 Victoria Embankment
London EC4Y 0DZ

An Hachette UK Company
www.hachette.co.uk
www.hachettechildrens.co.uk

Printed in Italy

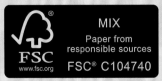

MIX
Paper from
responsible sources
FSC® C104740
FSC
www.fsc.org